Dr. Barbara Healing Bible

The Complete Guide to Barbara O'Neill's Herbal Remedies, Natural Medicine, and Teachings to Discover What the Big Pharma Doesn't Want You to Know

Michael Johnson

© Copyright 2024 - All rights reserved.

The content contained within this book may not be reproduced, duplicated or transmitted without direct written permission from the author or the publisher. Under no circumstances will any blame or legal responsibility be held against the publisher, or author, for any damages, reparation, or monetary loss due to the information contained within this book. Either **directly or indirectly.**

Legal Notice:

This book is copyright protected. This book is only for personal use. You cannot amend, distribute, sell, use, quote or paraphrase any part, or the content within this book, without the consent of the author or publisher.

Disclaimer Notice:

Please note the information contained within this document is for educational and entertainment purposes only. All effort has been executed to present accurate, up to date, and reliable, complete information. No warranties of any kind are declared or implied. Readers acknowledge that the author is not engaging in the rendering of legal, financial, medical or professional advice. The content within this book has been derived from various sources. Please consult a licensed professional before attempting any techniques outlined in this book.

By reading this document, the reader agrees that under no circumstances is the author responsible for any losses, direct or indirect, which are incurred as a result of the use of information contained within this document, including, but not limited to, errors, omissions, or inaccuracies.

Table of Contents

Introduction 5

Chapter 1: 7

Who is Barbara O'Neill 7

Chapter 2: 14

Foundations of Health According to Barbara 14

Chapter 3: 22

Diet and Nutrition 22

Chapter 4: 31

Natural Remedies and Prevention 31

Chapter 5: 39

Managing Stress and Mental Health 39

Chapter 6: 47

Physical Exercise for Health 47

Chapter 7: 56

Addressing Common Ailments and Diseases 56

Chapter 8: 66

Specific Remedies for Common Conditions 66

Chapter 9: 75

Success Stories 75

Chapter 10: 81

Building Your Wellness Routine 81

Glossary of Terms 90

Summary of Key Principles 94

Encouragement for the Journey Towards Health 97

Conclusion 101

Introduction

Welcome to the journey towards a healthier and more harmonious life with "Dr. Barbara". This book is not merely a tribute to the wisdom and legacy of Barbara O'Neill, a renowned educator in the field of natural health; it is also a practical guide aimed at transforming your understanding and practice of wellness. Through the pages that follow, we invite you to explore the teachings of a woman who has dedicated her life to demonstrating how nature can be our most powerful ally in the quest for health.

In a world where conventional medicine often takes precedence, Barbara's philosophy reminds us of the importance of getting back to basics. From balanced nutrition and the significance of physical exercise to natural remedies and stress management strategies, this book is an invitation to rediscover the simple truths that can guide us towards optimal health.

But "Dr. Barbara" is more than just a collection of health advice. It is a story of transformation and hope. Through touching testimonials and success stories, you will see how the principles shared in this book have the power to change lives. Whether you are looking to improve your overall health or are facing specific challenges, you will find practical advice and inspiration to take concrete steps towards wellness.

This book is also a reminder that we are not alone in our journey towards health. Each chapter will guide you, like a friendly hand, showing you how to implement positive changes that can be both simple and transformative. From strategies for better nutrition to discovering natural remedies for common ailments, "Dr. Barbara" is a valuable resource for anyone wishing to take control of their health in a natural and informed way.

Embark on this journey with us, armed with curiosity and openness, ready to explore a health approach that celebrates life in all its forms. "Dr. Barbara" is not just a book; it is a step towards a fuller, richer life in harmony with the natural world.

With every page you turn, we wish you not only to learn but to be inspired to make choices that nourish your body, mind, and spirit. Welcome to your new adventure towards health.

Chapter 1:

Who is Barbara O'Neill

Biography

Barbara O'Neill is an embodiment of dedication and passion in the field of natural health and wellness. A self-taught nutritionist and health educator, her journey into the realm of natural healing began from a genuine desire to help people achieve optimal health through simple, nature-aligned practices and lifestyle changes.

Born into a family that valued the principles of health and nutrition, Barbara's interest in natural remedies and preventive health care was sparked at an early age. Her academic path, rich with studies in the science of nutrition, anatomy, and the healing power of plants, laid a strong foundation for her future endeavors. However, it was her continuous self-education and unwavering commitment to understanding the human body's natural healing capabilities that truly defined her career.

Barbara's professional life has been characterized by a series of roles that reflect her diverse talents and her mission to educate others. She has served as a nutritionist, health educator, and motivational speaker, traveling extensively to share her knowledge. With an engaging and accessible approach, Barbara has inspired thousands to reconsider their lifestyle choices and embrace a more holistic approach to health.

Her teachings are not just theoretical. Barbara practices what she preaches, living a lifestyle that embodies her principles of health and wellness. This authentic living has earned her respect and credibility in the natural health community. Her work extends beyond personal consultations and seminars; Barbara has authored several books and produced educational videos that delve into various aspects of natural health, from diet and detoxification to stress management and disease prevention.

Barbara O'Neill is also known for her contributions to the Misty Mountain Health Retreat, where she has worked alongside her husband, offering wellness programs that integrate her teachings into practical, life-changing experiences for participants. This retreat reflects her holistic view of health, emphasizing the balance between physical, mental, and spiritual well-being.

Through her tireless work and dedication, Barbara O'Neill has become a beacon of hope and inspiration for those seeking to regain control of their health naturally. Her legacy is a testament to the power of education, passion, and the undying belief in the healing power of nature.

Professional Journey and Education

Barbara O'Neill's professional journey and educational background are testaments to her lifelong commitment to natural health and her pursuit of knowledge. Unlike traditional paths often trodden in the health sector, Barbara's story is one of exploration, self-education, and a deep-seated belief in the power of nature to heal.

Education

Barbara's formal education laid the groundwork for her expansive knowledge of natural health. Initially, she pursued studies in the sciences, which provided her with a critical understanding of human anatomy, physiology, and nutrition. However, Barbara's true education has been largely self-directed and experiential. Over the years, she has immersed herself in a wide array of subjects related to health and wellness, including but not limited to, naturopathy, herbal medicine, hydrotherapy, and the principles of holistic living.

This diverse and comprehensive self-education allowed Barbara to develop a unique perspective on health, one that sees the body as an interconnected system that can heal itself if given the right conditions and support. Her approach is deeply rooted in the belief that education about one's body and the natural world is paramount to achieving and maintaining health.

Professional Journey

Barbara O'Neill's professional journey is characterized by her dedication to teaching and her desire to make a tangible difference in people's lives. Starting her career in health education, Barbara quickly realized the impact of sharing knowledge and empowering individuals to take charge of their health. Her early work involved conducting seminars and workshops where she shared her insights on nutrition, the importance of detoxification, and the benefits of adopting a holistic lifestyle.

Her passion for teaching and her effectiveness as an educator led her to found and direct health retreats, most notably the Misty Mountain Health Retreat. Here, Barbara and her team offer programs designed to educate participants on natural health while providing them with the tools and experiences to implement lasting changes in their lives. These retreats encapsulate Barbara's holistic approach to health, combining nutritional advice, physical exercise, and mental and spiritual guidance.

Throughout her career, Barbara has also been an avid writer and content creator, producing numerous books, articles, and videos that cover a broad spectrum of health-related topics. These resources have made her teachings accessible to a global audience, extending her influence far beyond the confines of seminars and retreats.

Barbara O'Neill's professional journey is not just a career; it is a manifestation of her life's purpose. Through her education, writing, and hands-on work at health retreats, she has touched the lives of many, inspiring a return to natural living and the principles of self-care and wellness.

End of Professional Journey and Education Section

Barbara O'Neill's story exemplifies how passion, self-motivation, and a commitment to learning and teaching can lead to a fulfilling career that not only benefits oneself but also contributes positively to the lives of others.

Philosophy and Approach to Health

Barbara O'Neill's philosophy and approach to health are grounded in the belief that the body possesses an innate ability to heal itself, given the proper nourishment, care, and environment. This core belief has shaped her entire career and is evident in every aspect of her teachings. Her approach to health is holistic, emphasizing the interconnectedness of the mind, body, and spirit, and the importance of addressing all aspects of one's life to achieve true wellness.

Holistic Health as a Way of Life

For Barbara, health is not merely the absence of disease but a state of complete physical, mental, and social well-being. She advocates for a holistic approach to health, which considers the whole person and how they interact with their environment. This approach encourages a balanced lifestyle that includes a nutritious diet, regular physical activity, adequate rest, and positive social interactions.

Prevention Over Cure

A cornerstone of Barbara's philosophy is the emphasis on disease prevention rather than solely focusing on the cure. She believes in educating people about the root causes of illnesses and empowering them with the knowledge and tools to prevent these conditions. This preventive approach is centered around lifestyle modifications and natural remedies that support the body's healing processes.

The Healing Power of Nature

Barbara has a profound respect for the healing power of nature. She often emphasizes the importance of natural foods, herbs, and therapies in maintaining health and treating illnesses. According to her, nature provides us with everything we need to heal and thrive; it's simply a matter of understanding how to use these natural resources effectively.

Education as Empowerment

A key component of Barbara's approach is the empowerment through education. She dedicates a significant portion of her work to teaching people about their bodies, how they function, and how lifestyle choices affect health and well-being. Barbara believes that informed individuals are more likely to make healthy choices and take proactive steps towards maintaining their health.

Individualized Health Care

Recognizing that every person is unique, Barbara advocates for personalized health care plans that are tailored to the individual's specific needs, conditions, and lifestyle. She encourages people to listen to their bodies and adjust their health practices accordingly. This individualized approach ensures that health recommendations are not only effective but also sustainable in the long term.

Simplicity in Health

In an age of information overload and complex health trends, Barbara's teachings stand out for their simplicity and practicality. She demystifies health and wellness, making it accessible to everyone, regardless of their background or level of knowledge. Her message is clear: simple changes in diet, exercise, and mindset can have profound impacts on one's health.

Barbara O'Neill's philosophy and approach to health offer a refreshing perspective in a world often dominated by quick fixes and pharmaceutical solutions. Her emphasis on holistic health, prevention, natural remedies, and education not only inspires individuals to take control of their health but also promotes a deeper understanding of the natural world's role in our well-being. Through her work, Barbara continues to be a guiding light for those seeking a path to true health and vitality.

Chapter 2:

Foundations of Health According to Barbara

Importance of Natural Wellness

In the teachings of Barbara O'Neill, natural wellness occupies a central role, serving as the foundation upon which a healthy and fulfilling life is built. This concept of natural wellness is not just about the absence of illness; it's a holistic state of being that encompasses physical, mental, emotional, and spiritual health. Barbara's emphasis on natural wellness reflects her deep conviction that living in harmony with nature's principles is the key to achieving and maintaining optimal health.

The Essence of Natural Wellness

At the heart of natural wellness is the belief that the body is designed to maintain health and equilibrium, provided it's supported by a lifestyle that aligns with nature's laws. This includes eating whole, natural foods, ensuring adequate physical movement, getting sufficient rest, and managing stress effectively. By adhering to these simple yet profound principles, individuals can bolster their health naturally, reducing their reliance on medical interventions.

Nutrition as Nature Intended

Barbara places a strong emphasis on the power of nutrition in achieving natural wellness. She advocates for a diet rich in whole, plant-based foods that are minimally processed. These foods are packed with the nutrients needed to support the body's various functions and are more easily recognized and utilized by the body compared to synthetic supplements or heavily processed foods. By choosing foods that are as close to their natural state as possible, individuals can support their body's innate healing mechanisms.

The Healing Power of Water and Sunlight

Water and sunlight are also pivotal elements in Barbara's approach to natural wellness. Hydration plays a crucial role in maintaining health, as water is involved in nearly every bodily function. Similarly, sunlight provides essential vitamin D, which supports bone health, immune function, and mood regulation. Barbara encourages regular, moderate exposure to sunlight and the consumption of clean, pure water as simple yet effective practices for enhancing health.

The Importance of Physical Movement

Physical activity is another cornerstone of natural wellness. Barbara emphasizes that regular movement is vital for maintaining the health of the body and mind. Exercise improves circulation, boosts mood, supports detoxification, and enhances overall vitality. Whether it's walking, gardening, yoga, or any other form of activity that connects one with nature, incorporating regular physical movement into daily life is key to natural wellness.

Rest and Stress Management

Acknowledging the fast-paced and often stressful nature of modern life, Barbara underscores the importance of rest and stress management in achieving natural wellness. Quality sleep and relaxation techniques such as meditation or deep-breathing exercises are essential for allowing the body to repair, recover, and maintain a state of balance. Managing stress effectively is not only crucial for mental and emotional well-being but also has profound implications for physical health.

Connecting with Nature

Finally, Barbara O'Neill's concept of natural wellness involves a deep connection with the natural world. Spending time in nature, whether through outdoor activities, gardening, or simply taking a moment to appreciate the beauty of the natural environment, can have therapeutic effects on the mind and body. This connection not only enhances one's appreciation for the planet but also reinforces the importance of living in a way that is sustainable and respectful of the earth's resources.

Pillars of Health: Diet, Exercise, Water, Sunlight

In her teachings, Barbara O'Neill identifies four fundamental pillars of health that are essential for maintaining and enhancing our well-being: Diet, Exercise, Water, and Sunlight. Each of these pillars supports the body's natural ability to heal and maintain equilibrium. By focusing on these key areas, individuals can create a solid foundation for optimal health.

Diet: The Foundation of Vitality

A nutritious diet is at the heart of good health. Barbara emphasizes the importance of consuming a variety of whole, plant-based foods that are rich in vitamins, minerals, and antioxidants. These nutrients are crucial for the body's repair, growth, and maintenance processes. Foods such as fruits, vegetables, whole grains, nuts, and seeds provide the necessary fuel and building blocks for the body to function effectively. Processed foods, high in sugar and unhealthy fats, on the other hand, can contribute to inflammation and chronic diseases. A balanced diet, according to Barbara, is one that nourishes the body, supports its healing processes, and promotes vitality.

Exercise: Movement as Medicine

Regular physical activity is recognized as a cornerstone of good health. Exercise strengthens the heart and lungs, enhances muscle strength and flexibility, improves circulation, and helps control weight. Barbara advocates for incorporating exercise into daily life as a means to boost energy levels, improve mood, and reduce the risk of chronic diseases such as heart disease, diabetes, and obesity. Whether it's through walking, gardening, swimming, or practicing yoga, engaging in physical activities that one enjoys ensures sustainability and contributes to overall well-being.

Water: The Essence of Life

Water is vital for life and is involved in nearly every bodily function, including digestion, absorption, circulation, and excretion. It also plays a key role in regulating body temperature and maintaining electrolyte balance. Barbara stresses the importance of staying well-hydrated by drinking pure, clean water throughout the day. Adequate hydration supports the body's detoxification processes, improves skin health, and enhances cognitive function.

Sunlight: A Source of Energy and Health

Sunlight is essential for the production of vitamin D, a critical nutrient that supports bone health, immune function, and mood regulation. Barbara highlights the benefits of moderate sun exposure, recommending that individuals seek to spend a portion of their day outdoors in natural sunlight. Besides vitamin D production, sunlight exposure has been shown to improve sleep quality by regulating the body's circadian rhythm, reducing the risk of depression, and even lowering blood pressure.

Integrating the Pillars into Daily Life

Integrating these four pillars into daily life is a holistic approach that promotes natural wellness. Barbara suggests starting with small, manageable changes and gradually building upon them. For example, incorporating more whole foods into meals, taking short walks during the day, drinking a glass of water upon waking, and spending time outside in natural sunlight can all be simple starting points.

The synergy among diet, exercise, water, and sunlight creates a powerful foundation for health. Each pillar supports the others, contributing to a balanced and healthy lifestyle.

By focusing on these essential aspects of health, individuals can harness their body's inherent ability to heal and maintain optimal well-being.

Rest, Moderation, and Fresh Air

In addition to the core pillars of Diet, Exercise, Water, and Sunlight, Barbara O'Neill places significant emphasis on three equally important aspects of health and well-being: Rest, Moderation, and Fresh Air. These elements are vital for maintaining balance and supporting the body's natural healing processes.

Rest: Rejuvenation for Body and Mind

Rest is essential for health and vitality. It allows the body and mind to recover, repair, and rejuvenate. Barbara advocates for quality sleep and relaxation as foundational components of good health. Adequate rest is linked to improved concentration, memory, and mood; it also plays a critical role in immune function, metabolism, and the body's ability to heal.

Barbara emphasizes the importance of establishing a regular sleep routine, aiming for 7-9 hours of uninterrupted sleep per night. Creating a sleep-conducive environment, free from electronic devices and distractions, can enhance the quality of rest. Additionally, incorporating relaxation practices such as meditation, deep breathing, or gentle yoga before bedtime can help ease the transition into restful sleep.

Moderation: The Key to Balance

Moderation is a guiding principle in Barbara's approach to health. It applies to all areas of life, including diet, exercise, work, and leisure activities. The concept of moderation encourages a balanced lifestyle, avoiding extremes and fostering long-term sustainability.

Barbara teaches that overindulgence, even in healthy activities or foods, can lead to imbalance and health issues. For example, excessive exercise can increase the risk of injury, and overeating healthy foods can lead to digestive discomfort. By practicing moderation, individuals can enjoy a variety of foods and activities while maintaining their health and well-being.

Fresh Air: Vital for Health

Fresh air is another cornerstone of natural wellness. Breathing clean, fresh air is vital for maintaining good health, as it supplies the body with oxygen while helping to remove waste gases and toxins through exhalation. Barbara underscores the importance of spending time outdoors in natural environments to take advantage of the quality air and the overall health benefits it provides.

Regular exposure to fresh air is associated with improved lung function, enhanced immune system performance, and a boost in mood and energy levels. Barbara encourages outdoor activities, such as walking, gardening, or simply sitting in a park, as effective ways to increase fresh air intake. Ventilating living spaces by opening windows and minimizing the use of air conditioners can also improve indoor air quality, contributing to better health.

Integrating Rest, Moderation, and Fresh Air into Daily Life

Integrating rest, moderation, and fresh air into daily life involves making conscious choices and adjustments to one's lifestyle. Establishing a consistent sleep schedule, practicing mindful eating and activity, and prioritizing time outdoors are all strategies that support these health components. By doing so, individuals can enhance their physical, mental, and emotional well-being.

Rest, Moderation, and Fresh Air, along with the foundational pillars of Diet, Exercise, Water, and Sunlight, form a comprehensive approach to health and wellness. Barbara O'Neill's emphasis on these principles highlights the importance of a holistic and balanced lifestyle. Adopting practices that support these aspects of health can lead to significant improvements in overall well-being, vitality, and happiness.

Chapter 3:

Diet and Nutrition

Principles of a Healthy Diet

In the teachings of Barbara O'Neill, the principles of a healthy diet are pivotal for achieving optimal health and wellness. Through her holistic approach to nutrition, Barbara emphasizes the importance of adopting dietary habits that support the body's natural processes and promote healing. The principles outlined below serve as a foundation for nourishing the body, enhancing vitality, and preventing disease.

Whole Foods Over Processed Foods

One of the cornerstones of Barbara's dietary philosophy is the emphasis on whole foods. These are foods that are consumed as close to their natural state as possible, minimally processed and free from artificial additives. Whole foods include fresh fruits and vegetables, whole grains, nuts, seeds, and legumes. They are rich in essential nutrients, fiber, and phytochemicals that support bodily functions and protect against chronic diseases.

Plant-Based Nutrition

Barbara advocates for a diet that is predominantly plant-based. Plant-based diets are centered around plants, including vegetables, fruits, grains, nuts, seeds, and legumes, and are known for their health benefits. This doesn't necessarily mean a strictly vegetarian or vegan diet, but rather a diet in which plant foods make up the majority of the intake. Such a diet is associated with lower risks of heart disease, hypertension, diabetes, and certain types of cancer.

Adequate Hydration

Proper hydration is vital for maintaining health. Water plays a key role in every bodily function, including digestion, absorption, circulation, and temperature regulation.

Barbara stresses the importance of drinking sufficient pure water daily to support these functions, enhance detoxification, and promote skin health. The recommendation often cited is to drink at least eight 8-ounce glasses of water a day, although individual needs may vary based on factors like activity level and climate.

Moderation and Balance

Eating in moderation is a principle that Barbara emphasizes for maintaining a healthy diet. This involves consuming a variety of foods in appropriate quantities to avoid excesses or deficiencies in nutrient intake. It's about finding balance and listening to the body's cues for hunger and fullness, ensuring that food intake supports health without leading to weight gain or nutrient imbalances.

Limiting Refined Sugars and Processed Foods

A significant aspect of a healthy diet involves minimizing the intake of refined sugars and processed foods. These foods are often high in calories but low in nutritional value, and their consumption can lead to weight gain, insulin resistance, and other health issues. Barbara advises limiting foods and beverages high in added sugars and opting for natural sweeteners in moderation.

Incorporating Healthy Fats

Healthy fats are an essential part of a balanced diet. Contrary to the outdated belief that all fats are bad, Barbara highlights the importance of including sources of healthy fats, such as avocados, nuts, seeds, and cold-pressed oils like olive oil. These fats are crucial for brain health, hormone production, and the absorption of fat-soluble vitamins.

Listening to Your Body

Finally, Barbara encourages individuals to listen to their bodies and adjust their diets according to their needs, preferences, and reactions to different foods. Recognizing that each person is unique, she advocates for a personalized approach to nutrition that respects the body's signals and promotes overall well-being.

The principles of a healthy diet as outlined by Barbara O'Neill offer a comprehensive guide to eating well and living in harmony with nature's design for our bodies. By adopting these dietary practices, individuals can support their health naturally, reduce the risk of chronic diseases, and enhance their quality of life.

Foods to Favor and Avoid

In the context of Barbara O'Neill's teachings on natural health, making informed choices about what to eat is fundamental. This section outlines the types of foods she advocates incorporating into your diet for optimal health, as well as those to minimize or avoid. Embracing this approach can lead to significant improvements in overall well-being, energy levels, and disease prevention.

Foods to Favor

Whole Grains: Choose whole, unrefined grains such as brown rice, quinoa, oats, and barley. These grains provide essential nutrients, including fiber, vitamins, and minerals, that support digestion and can help maintain stable blood sugar levels.

Fruits and Vegetables: Emphasize a variety of fresh or frozen fruits and vegetables. They are rich in antioxidants, vitamins, minerals, and fiber, which are essential for maintaining good health and preventing chronic diseases. Aim for a rainbow of colors to ensure a broad intake of nutrients.

Legumes: Beans, lentils, and chickpeas are excellent plant-based protein sources. They also offer fiber, iron, and phytonutrients that support bodily functions and can help reduce cholesterol levels.

Nuts and Seeds: Almonds, walnuts, flaxseeds, chia seeds, and hemp seeds are good sources of healthy fats, protein, and fiber. They can contribute to heart health and provide essential fatty acids that the body cannot produce on its own.

Healthy Fats: Incorporate sources of healthy fats, such as avocados, olive oil, and coconut oil. These fats are crucial for brain function, hormone production, and the absorption of vitamins A, D, E, and K.

Herbs and Spices: Use a variety of herbs and spices to flavor your food naturally. Many herbs and spices, including turmeric, ginger, and garlic, have anti-inflammatory properties and health benefits.

Hydration: Prioritize pure water for hydration. Herbal teas and freshly squeezed vegetable juices can also be beneficial, providing hydration along with vitamins and minerals.

Foods to Avoid

Processed and Junk Foods: Limit or eliminate foods that are highly processed or high in added sugars and unhealthy fats. These include fast food, sweets, sodas, and snack foods, which can contribute to inflammation, weight gain, and chronic diseases.

Refined Carbohydrates: Avoid white bread, pasta, and other refined grains that have been stripped of their fiber and nutrients. These foods can lead to spikes in blood sugar levels and have little nutritional value.

Excessive Caffeine and Alcohol: While moderate consumption may be acceptable for some individuals, excessive intake of caffeine and alcohol can negatively affect health, disrupting sleep patterns and contributing to dehydration and nutrient imbalances.

Artificial Additives: Steer clear of artificial colors, flavors, sweeteners, and preservatives. These chemicals can have adverse effects on health and well-being, and some are linked to increased health risks.

Trans Fats and Hydrogenated Oils: Trans fats, found in some margarines, processed foods, and baked goods, should be avoided due to their association with increased heart disease risk.

High-Sodium Foods: Limit foods high in sodium, such as processed meats, canned soups, and fast foods, to reduce blood pressure and risk of cardiovascular disease.

Adopting a diet that favors whole, nutrient-dense foods while avoiding processed foods and unhealthy fats aligns with Barbara O'Neill's principles for maintaining health and vitality. By making conscious food choices, individuals can support their body's natural healing processes and enjoy a higher quality of life.

Tips for Transitioning to a Healthier Diet

Adopting a healthier diet can seem daunting at first, especially if you're used to eating processed foods, high amounts of sugar, or fast food. However, Barbara O'Neill emphasizes that transitioning to a more nutritious diet is a journey that doesn't have to be overwhelming. Here are practical tips inspired by her teachings that can help you gradually shift towards healthier eating habits.

Start Small

Begin with small, manageable changes rather than overhauling your diet overnight. For example, start by incorporating one additional serving of vegetables into your meals each day or swapping out your morning sugary cereal for a whole grain alternative with fresh fruit. Small changes can add up to significant health benefits over time.

Plan Your Meals

Meal planning can help you make healthier choices and avoid the temptation of fast food or processed meals. Spend some time each week planning your meals and snacks. This can also help you save time and reduce food waste.

Cook at Home

Cooking at home gives you control over the ingredients and allows you to make healthier versions of your favorite dishes. Experiment with recipes that use whole, unprocessed foods. Cooking can be a rewarding and creative activity that contributes to your overall well-being.

Increase Plant-Based Foods

Gradually increase the amount of plant-based foods in your diet. Aim to fill half your plate with vegetables at lunch and dinner. Explore plant-based sources of protein like beans, lentils, and tofu. Incorporating more plant-based foods can lead to increased fiber intake, essential nutrients, and a variety of health benefits.

Listen to Your Body

Pay attention to how different foods make you feel. Notice any changes in your energy levels, digestion, or overall well-being as you adjust your diet. Listening to your body can guide you toward foods that nourish and satisfy you.

Stay Hydrated

Sometimes thirst is mistaken for hunger. Ensure you're drinking enough water throughout the day. Keeping hydrated can aid digestion, improve skin health, and help control hunger.

Find Support

Making dietary changes can be easier with support from friends, family, or a community with similar health goals. Share recipes, cook together, or update each other on your progress. Support can provide motivation and make the transition more enjoyable.

Be Patient and Kind to Yourself

Transitioning to a healthier diet is a process, and it's normal to have setbacks. Be patient and kind to yourself. Celebrate your successes, and don't be too hard on yourself if you slip up. Remember, the goal is long-term health and well-being.

Educate Yourself

Knowledge is empowering. Learn about the health benefits of different foods, and stay informed about nutrition. Understanding why certain foods are beneficial can motivate you to make healthier choices.

Gradual Replacement Strategy

Instead of cutting out all "unhealthy" foods at once, try gradually replacing them with healthier alternatives. For instance, if you drink a lot of sugary beverages, start by

replacing one drink per day with water or herbal tea. Over time, these healthier choices will become part of your routine.

Chapter 4:

Natural Remedies and Prevention

The Use of Herbs in Healing

The use of herbs in healing is a time-honored tradition that dates back thousands of years. Herbs, with their complex array of phytochemicals, offer a natural and holistic approach to health and wellness. Barbara O'Neill, a staunch advocate for natural health, emphasizes the importance of understanding and utilizing the healing properties of herbs. This chapter explores how herbs can be integrated into daily life to support health, prevent illness, and treat various conditions.

Understanding Herbs

Herbs are plants with specific therapeutic properties. They can be used in various forms, including teas, tinctures, capsules, powders, and topical applications. Each herb has its unique profile of active compounds that contribute to its healing effects. When selecting herbs for healing, it's crucial to choose high-quality, organic products to ensure their efficacy and safety.

Common Healing Herbs and Their Uses

Several herbs have been widely recognized for their health benefits. Here are a few examples, along with their traditional uses:

- **Chamomile:** Known for its calming effects, chamomile is often used to relieve stress, promote relaxation, and improve sleep quality. It also has anti-inflammatory properties, making it beneficial for digestive discomfort.
- **Ginger:** With its potent anti-inflammatory and antioxidant effects, ginger is commonly used to alleviate nausea, support digestion, and reduce pain, particularly related to arthritis and menstrual discomfort.

- **Turmeric:** Curcumin, the active compound in turmeric, has powerful anti-inflammatory and antioxidant properties. Turmeric is often used to support joint health, improve digestion, and boost the immune system.
- **Peppermint:** Peppermint is renowned for its ability to soothe digestive issues, such as irritable bowel syndrome (IBS), gas, and bloating. It also has analgesic properties, making it useful for relieving headaches.
- **Echinacea:** Often used to prevent and treat the common cold, echinacea has been shown to boost the immune system and reduce inflammation.
- **Lavender:** Lavender is well-loved for its calming and relaxing scent. It is used to alleviate stress, improve sleep, and, in topical applications, treat skin irritations and wounds

Incorporating Herbs into Your Health Regimen

To effectively incorporate herbs into your health regimen, consider the following tips:

- Consult with a Professional: Before adding new herbs to your routine, especially if you have existing health conditions or are taking medication, consult with a healthcare professional knowledgeable about herbal medicine.
- Start Slowly: Begin with one herb at a time to monitor its effects on your body. This approach allows you to determine how you respond to each herb and adjust accordingly.
- Educate Yourself: Learn about the herbs you're interested in, including their uses, potential side effects, and interactions with other herbs or medications.
- Listen to Your Body: Pay attention to how your body reacts to different herbs. What works for one person may not work for another, so it's essential to find what works best for you.

Herbs offer a natural and effective way to support health and treat various ailments. By understanding the healing properties of herbs and how to use them responsibly, you can harness the power of nature to enhance your well-being. As with any health intervention, it's important to approach herbal medicine with caution, respect, and knowledge.

Hydrotherapy and Its Benefits

Hydrotherapy, or water therapy, is a practice that involves the use of water in various forms and temperatures to promote health and healing. This ancient technique, which has been utilized for centuries across different cultures, remains a vital component of natural health care. Barbara O'Neill advocates for the inclusion of hydrotherapy in a holistic health regimen, highlighting its versatility and numerous health benefits. This section delves into the principles of hydrotherapy and the wide range of benefits it offers.

Principles of Hydrotherapy

The foundation of hydrotherapy lies in its ability to manipulate the body's response to hot and cold stimuli. The application of water at different temperatures can cause the body to react in specific ways, promoting healing and wellness. Warm water can relax muscles, increase blood circulation, and soothe nerves, while cold water can invigorate the body, reduce inflammation, and stimulate the immune system.

Common Hydrotherapy Treatments

- Contrast Showers: Alternating between hot and cold water during a shower to improve circulation, invigorate the skin, and stimulate the immune system.
- Warm Baths: Soaking in warm water to relieve muscle tension, reduce stress, and promote relaxation. Adding Epsom salts or essential oils can enhance the therapeutic effects.

- Cold Compresses: Applying a cold compress to reduce acute inflammation, alleviate pain, or lower body temperature during fever.
- Steam Baths/Saunas: Using steam to encourage sweating, which helps detoxify the body and relax the muscles.
- Water Exercise: Performing exercises in a pool to reduce the strain on joints while providing resistance for muscle strengthening.

Benefits of Hydrotherapy

- Pain Relief: Hydrotherapy can alleviate pain associated with conditions such as arthritis, fibromyalgia, and low back pain through muscle relaxation and improved circulation.
- Stress Reduction: Water has a calming effect on the mind and body, reducing stress and promoting a sense of well-being.
- Improved Circulation: The use of hot and cold water can stimulate blood flow, enhancing the delivery of oxygen and nutrients to tissues while aiding in the removal of waste products.
- Enhanced Immune Function: Alternating between hot and cold water can stimulate the immune system, potentially reducing the frequency and severity of colds and other infections.
- Detoxification: Sweat induced by steam baths or saunas can help eliminate toxins from the body, supporting overall health.
- Muscle and Joint Health: Hydrotherapy can relieve muscle tension and stiffness, support joint mobility, and reduce the symptoms of arthritis and other musculoskeletal conditions.
- Incorporating Hydrotherapy into Your Routine

Incorporating hydrotherapy into your health regimen can be simple and does not necessarily require expensive equipment or visits to a spa. Many hydrotherapy techniques, such as contrast showers, warm baths, and cold compresses, can be easily practiced at home. Listening to your body and adjusting the temperature and duration of treatments to your comfort and health goals is essential.

Natural Detox Techniques

In a world where exposure to toxins is an everyday occurrence—through the environment, food, and lifestyle choices—detoxification processes hold a significant place in maintaining health. Barbara O'Neill emphasizes the importance of supporting the body's natural detoxification pathways to enhance overall wellness. This section outlines various natural detox techniques that can be incorporated into a holistic health regimen to aid the body in eliminating toxins and improving health.

1. Hydration

Water is essential for detoxification. It aids in flushing toxins out of the body through the kidneys, helps maintain a healthy digestive system to eliminate waste, and supports optimal blood circulation. Drinking adequate amounts of clean, filtered water throughout the day is a simple yet effective detox strategy.

2. Diet Focused on Whole Foods

A diet rich in whole, organic foods plays a crucial role in detoxification. Foods high in antioxidants, fiber, vitamins, and minerals support the liver and other detox organs. Incorporating a variety of fruits, vegetables, whole grains, nuts, seeds, and legumes into your diet can enhance the body's natural detox processes.

3. Regular Physical Activity

Exercise is not just vital for overall health but also for promoting detoxification. Physical activity increases blood circulation and promotes sweat, helping to eliminate toxins through the skin. Regular exercise can also boost the lymphatic system, another critical component of the body's natural detox mechanisms.

4. Saunas and Steam Baths

Using a sauna or steam bath can encourage the body to sweat out toxins. The heat from saunas and steam baths raises the body's core temperature, simulating a fever—a natural mechanism for fighting infections and detoxifying. This process can aid in eliminating heavy metals and other toxins through the skin.

5. Dry Skin Brushing

Dry skin brushing is a technique that involves using a dry brush to gently brush the skin in a particular pattern, typically towards the heart. This method helps stimulate the lymphatic system, which plays a key role in removing waste and toxins from the body. Dry skin brushing also removes dead skin cells, improving skin health and appearance.

6. Herbal Detox Teas

Certain herbs have detoxifying properties and can support the body's natural detox processes when consumed as teas. Herbs such as dandelion, milk thistle, green tea, and nettle have been traditionally used to support liver function, improve kidney health, and aid in digestion.

7. Adequate Sleep

Sleep is crucial for the body's healing and detoxification processes. During sleep, the brain's glymphatic system becomes active, clearing out waste from the central nervous system. Ensuring adequate, restful sleep supports the body's natural detoxification processes and promotes overall health.

Incorporating natural detox techniques into your lifestyle can support the body's inherent ability to cleanse itself, leading to improved health and vitality. While these methods can enhance the body's detoxification processes, it's also important to reduce exposure to toxins whenever possible. As with any health regimen, it's advisable to consult with a healthcare professional, especially if you have underlying health conditions, to ensure that detoxification practices are safe and suitable for your individual health needs.

Chapter 5:

Managing Stress and Mental Health

Relaxation and Meditation Techniques

In the holistic approach to health, mental and emotional well-being are as important as physical health. Stress and anxiety not only affect one's quality of life but can also have profound effects on physical health, including increased risk for chronic diseases, weakened immune system, and impaired digestion. Barbara O'Neill emphasizes the importance of incorporating relaxation and meditation techniques into daily life to nurture mental and emotional balance. This section explores various practices that can help reduce stress, enhance emotional resilience, and promote a sense of inner peace.

Deep Breathing Techniques

Deep breathing is a simple yet powerful relaxation technique. It helps lower stress levels, reduce blood pressure, and improve oxygen delivery to the body. One popular method is the 4-7-8 technique, where you inhale deeply for 4 seconds, hold the breath for 7 seconds, and exhale slowly for 8 seconds. This practice can be done anywhere and anytime you feel stressed.

Guided Imagery

Guided imagery involves using your imagination to visualize a peaceful and calming scene or environment. This method engages the mind in a focused manner, diverting it from stress-inducing thoughts and promoting relaxation. You can find guided imagery scripts online or listen to recordings to help guide your visualization.

Progressive Muscle Relaxation (PMR)

Progressive muscle relaxation involves tensing and then slowly releasing each muscle group in the body, starting from the toes and moving upwards. This technique helps identify areas of tension and promotes overall relaxation. PMR is particularly beneficial for those who experience stress-related muscle tension.

Meditation

Meditation is a practice of focusing the mind on a particular object, thought, or activity to achieve a mentally clear and emotionally calm state. There are various forms of meditation, including mindfulness meditation, which involves paying attention to the present moment without judgment. Regular meditation has been shown to reduce stress, improve concentration, and enhance overall well-being.

Yoga and Tai Chi

Yoga and Tai Chi are practices that combine physical postures, breathing exercises, and meditation to promote relaxation and improve health. Both practices are effective in reducing stress, improving flexibility and balance, and enhancing mental clarity. Many community centers and gyms offer classes for all skill levels.

Journaling

Writing in a journal can be a therapeutic way to express thoughts and feelings, reflect on experiences, and identify sources of stress. Journaling can help process emotions and provide an outlet for releasing pent-up feelings, leading to greater emotional well-being.

Spending Time in Nature

Being in nature, whether it's a walk in the park, gardening, or simply sitting outside, can have a calming effect on the mind and body. Natural settings can reduce stress, improve mood, and increase feelings of connectedness and well-being.

The Importance of Sleep

Sleep is a fundamental component of overall health and well-being, deeply intertwined with both physical and mental health. Barbara O'Neill emphasizes that adequate, quality sleep is essential not just for rest and recuperation, but as a cornerstone of a holistic approach to health. This section delves into the critical role sleep plays in maintaining health, the consequences of sleep deprivation, and strategies to improve sleep quality.

The Role of Sleep in Health

Sleep serves multiple vital functions for the body and mind. Physiologically, it allows the body to repair and regenerate tissues, build bone and muscle, and strengthen the immune system. Neurologically, sleep is crucial for the consolidation of memories, learning, and emotional regulation. It also plays a significant role in regulating metabolism, appetite, and the risk of chronic diseases such as obesity, diabetes, and cardiovascular disease.

Consequences of Inadequate Sleep

Chronic sleep deprivation can have severe implications for health and well-being. Physically, it can lead to increased risk of chronic conditions, impaired immune function, and decreased life expectancy. Mentally, lack of sleep can contribute to cognitive impairments, memory issues, increased stress response, anxiety, and depression. Moreover, sleep deprivation can negatively affect emotional stability and the ability to cope with stress.

Strategies for Improving Sleep Quality

Improving sleep quality is within reach through adopting healthy sleep habits and creating an environment conducive to sleep. Barbara O'Neill recommends several strategies to enhance sleep:

- Establish a Regular Sleep Schedule: Going to bed and waking up at the same time every day helps regulate your body's internal clock and improve the quality of sleep.
- Create a Restful Environment: Ensure your bedroom is quiet, dark, and at a comfortable temperature. Invest in a good quality mattress and pillows to support a restful night's sleep.
- Limit Exposure to Screens Before Bedtime: The blue light emitted by screens can interfere with the production of melatonin, the hormone that signals your body it's time to sleep. Try to avoid screens at least an hour before bedtime.
- Mindful Eating and Drinking: Avoid heavy or large meals, caffeine, and alcohol before bedtime, as they can disrupt sleep.
- Relaxation Techniques: Incorporate relaxation practices such as reading, taking a warm bath, meditation, or deep breathing exercises before bed to help signal to your body that it's time to wind down.
- Physical Activity: Regular physical activity can help you fall asleep faster and enjoy deeper sleep, but try not to exercise too close to bedtime, as it might energize you.
- Manage Stress: Addressing daytime stressors and learning stress management techniques can improve sleep quality. Consider practices like journaling, time management strategies, and relaxation techniques to manage stress effectively.

Sleep is not merely a passive state of rest, but an active and integral part of our health and well-being. By prioritizing sleep and adopting healthy sleep habits, individuals can support their body's natural healing processes, enhance cognitive function, and improve emotional resilience. Recognizing the importance of sleep and taking steps to improve sleep quality can lead to significant improvements in quality of life and overall health.

Tips for a Healthy Mind

Maintaining a healthy mind is as crucial as taking care of our physical health. Mental and emotional well-being influences how we think, feel, and act, impacting our overall quality of life. Barbara O'Neill stresses the importance of nurturing our mental health through holistic practices that balance the mind, body, and spirit. This section offers practical tips for cultivating a healthy mind, fostering resilience, and enhancing emotional well-being.

1. Practice Mindfulness and Meditation

Mindfulness and meditation are powerful tools for maintaining mental health. They help center thoughts, calm the mind, and reduce stress and anxiety. By focusing on the present moment and observing thoughts and emotions without judgment, one can achieve a state of inner peace and clarity.

2. Cultivate Positive Relationships

Social connections are vital for emotional well-being. Cultivate relationships with people who support and uplift you. Quality social interactions can provide a sense of belonging and help reduce feelings of loneliness and isolation.

3. Engage in Regular Physical Activity

Exercise is not only beneficial for physical health but also for mental health. It releases endorphins, which have natural stress-relieving and mood-boosting effects. Find a physical activity you enjoy, whether it's walking, cycling, yoga, or dancing, and incorporate it into your routine.

4. Prioritize Sleep

Adequate sleep is essential for a healthy mind. Sleep helps to consolidate memories, process emotions, and rejuvenate the brain. Establish a regular sleep schedule and create a relaxing bedtime routine to improve sleep quality.

5. Set Realistic Goals

Setting and achieving goals can provide a sense of accomplishment and purpose. Start with small, achievable objectives and gradually work towards larger goals. Celebrate your successes along the way to boost your self-esteem and motivation.

6. Limit Screen Time

Excessive screen time, especially on social media, can negatively impact mental health. It can lead to comparison, dissatisfaction, and increased stress. Set boundaries for screen use and take regular breaks to disconnect and engage in real-world activities.

7. Learn New Skills

Learning new skills or hobbies can be mentally stimulating and rewarding. It can also provide a sense of achievement and improve self-confidence. Whether it's learning a musical instrument, a new language, or a craft, engaging in new activities can enrich your life and expand your horizons.

8. Practice Gratitude

Focusing on gratitude can shift your perspective and reduce stress. Take time each day to reflect on things you are thankful for, no matter how small. Keeping a gratitude journal can help you acknowledge and appreciate the positive aspects of your life.

9. Seek Professional Help When Needed

It's important to recognize when you need help and to seek professional support. If you're experiencing persistent feelings of sadness, anxiety, or other mental health concerns, talking to a counselor, psychologist, or psychiatrist can provide relief and guidance.

10. Embrace Nature

Spending time in nature has been shown to reduce stress, improve mood, and enhance mental clarity. Make time to go outside, whether for a walk in the park, gardening, or simply sitting in a natural setting, to reconnect with the natural world.

Chapter 6:

Physical Exercise for Health

Benefits of Regular Physical Activity

Regular physical activity is a cornerstone of a healthy lifestyle, playing a crucial role in promoting longevity and improving quality of life. Barbara O'Neill emphasizes the importance of integrating consistent exercise into our daily routines to harness the myriad benefits it offers for both body and mind. This section explores the extensive advantages of regular physical activity, underscoring its significance in achieving holistic health and well-being.

1. Enhances Cardiovascular Health

Regular exercise strengthens the heart and improves circulation, which reduces the risk of heart disease and stroke, leading causes of premature death worldwide. Activities like walking, cycling, and swimming increase heart rate, promoting efficient blood flow and lowering blood pressure.

2. Supports Weight Management

Physical activity, especially when combined with a balanced diet, is a key factor in maintaining a healthy weight and preventing obesity. Exercise burns calories, builds muscle, and boosts metabolism, making it easier to achieve and maintain weight loss goals.

3. Improves Muscular and Skeletal Health

Strength training and weight-bearing exercises enhance muscle strength, flexibility, and bone density. This can help prevent the loss of muscle mass and bone density that occurs with aging, reducing the risk of osteoporosis, fractures, and sarcopenia.

4. Boosts Mental Health

Exercise releases endorphins, often referred to as the body's natural mood lifters. Regular physical activity can alleviate symptoms of depression and anxiety, enhance mood, reduce stress, and improve sleep quality, contributing to overall mental and emotional well-being.

5. Enhances Cognitive Function

Studies suggest that regular physical activity can improve cognitive function, slow cognitive decline, and reduce the risk of developing neurodegenerative diseases such as Alzheimer's. Exercise increases blood flow to the brain, supports neuroplasticity, and may help grow new brain cells.

6. Supports Healthy Aging

Engaging in regular physical activity can delay the onset of chronic diseases and disabilities associated with aging, promoting independence and a higher quality of life in later years. Active individuals tend to have a longer lifespan and a better overall quality of life compared to those who are sedentary.

7. Improves Immune Function

Moderate-intensity exercise has been shown to boost the immune system, helping the body fight off infections and diseases. Regular physical activity promotes good circulation, which allows immune cells to move more efficiently throughout the body.

8. Increases Energy Levels

Regular exercise can increase stamina and reduce feelings of fatigue. By improving the efficiency of the cardiovascular system, physical activity ensures that oxygen and nutrients are effectively delivered to tissues, enhancing overall energy levels.

9. Promotes Better Sleep

Physical activity can help regulate sleep patterns and improve the quality of sleep. Engaging in regular exercise, particularly in the morning or afternoon, can deepen sleep and make it easier to fall asleep at night.

10. Fosters Social Connections

Many forms of exercise, such as group fitness classes, sports teams, and community events, provide opportunities to meet new people and build social networks. Social interactions associated with physical activity can enhance feelings of belonging and support overall mental health.

Exercises Recommended by Barbara

Barbara O'Neill, with her holistic approach to health and wellness, advocates for a variety of physical activities that cater to different fitness levels, interests, and health goals. Her recommendations emphasize the importance of incorporating exercises that not only improve physical health but also contribute to mental and emotional well-being. This section outlines a range of exercises that Barbara suggests for a balanced and comprehensive fitness routine.

1. Walking

Barbara often highlights walking as one of the most natural and accessible forms of exercise. It's suitable for people of all fitness levels and can be easily incorporated into daily routines. Walking improves cardiovascular health, aids in weight management, and can be a meditative practice that helps clear the mind and reduce stress.

2. Gardening

Gardening is another activity recommended for its physical and mental health benefits. It involves various movements that strengthen the body, such as bending, lifting, and digging, providing a moderate physical workout. Gardening also offers therapeutic benefits, including stress reduction and improved mood, due to its connection with nature and the outdoors.

3. Swimming

Swimming is praised for being a low-impact, whole-body workout that is particularly beneficial for individuals with joint issues or arthritis. It strengthens the cardiovascular system, tones muscles, and improves flexibility without putting strain on the joints, making it an ideal exercise for all ages and fitness levels.

4. Cycling

Cycling, whether outdoor or stationary, is an effective cardiovascular exercise that can help build endurance, strengthen leg muscles, and aid in weight loss. It's also low-impact on the joints and can be a fun way to explore the outdoors or enjoy a group exercise class.

5. Yoga

Yoga is recommended for its ability to improve flexibility, strength, and balance, as well as for its mental health benefits. The practice of yoga incorporates postures, breathing exercises, and meditation, helping to reduce stress, improve concentration, and promote a sense of inner peace.

6. Strength Training

Barbara advises incorporating strength training into regular exercise routines to build muscle, boost metabolism, and support bone health. Strength training can be adjusted to suit various fitness levels and goals, using bodyweight exercises, free weights, or resistance bands.

7. Tai Chi

Tai Chi is a gentle form of martial arts known for its health benefits, including improving balance, reducing stress, and enhancing mental focus. Its slow, deliberate movements make it an accessible exercise for older adults and those looking for a low-impact physical activity.

8. Pilates

Pilates focuses on core strength, flexibility, and overall body conditioning. This exercise is recommended for improving posture, muscle tone, and balance, as well as for rehabilitation purposes. Pilates can be modified to cater to different fitness levels and can be practiced with or without equipment.

Barbara O'Neill advocates for a holistic approach to fitness that incorporates a variety of exercises to benefit the body and mind. By engaging in activities like walking, gardening, swimming, cycling, yoga, strength training, Tai Chi, and Pilates, individuals can enjoy a comprehensive fitness routine that supports overall health, well-being, and longevity. The key is to find activities that you enjoy and can commit to regularly, fostering a healthy and active lifestyle.

How to Incorporate More Movement into Daily Life

In today's sedentary world, finding ways to incorporate more movement into our daily routines is crucial for maintaining health and promoting longevity. Barbara O'Neill emphasizes that regular physical activity should not be confined to structured exercise sessions alone. Instead, it's about integrating movement throughout the day to reduce sedentary behavior and enhance overall well-being. This section offers practical strategies for incorporating more physical activity into your daily life, ensuring that staying active becomes a natural and enjoyable part of your routine.

1. Take Short Walking Breaks

Make it a habit to take short walking breaks throughout the day, especially if you have a desk job. A brief 5 to 10-minute walk every hour can improve circulation, boost energy levels, and reduce the health risks associated with prolonged sitting.

2. Use Active Transportation

Whenever possible, opt for active modes of transportation such as walking, biking, or using public transport (which often involves walking to stations or stops). This not only contributes to your daily physical activity but also benefits the environment.

3. Stand More

Incorporate standing into activities where you would normally sit. Use a standing desk at work or take phone calls standing up. Standing burns more calories than sitting and can help reduce the risk of chronic diseases.

4. Take the Stairs

Choosing the stairs over elevators or escalators is an easy way to increase your heart rate and strengthen your legs. It's a simple change that can make a significant difference in your daily physical activity levels.

5. Turn Chores into Exercise

Household chores can be an excellent source of physical activity. Activities like vacuuming, gardening, and cleaning require bending, lifting, and stretching, all of which contribute to your daily movement quota.

6. Schedule Active Outings

Plan activities with friends and family that involve movement, such as hiking, biking, or playing a sport together. This not only makes exercise more enjoyable but also helps build a supportive community around physical activity.

7. Incorporate Exercise into Leisure Time

Instead of watching TV or browsing the internet during your leisure time, consider engaging in a physical activity you enjoy. This could be anything from dancing to yoga or even a simple walk in the park.

8. Practice Micro-Workouts

Micro-workouts involve short bursts of high-intensity exercises performed at various times throughout the day. Examples include doing a set of push-ups, squats, or lunges during a break. These can be highly effective in increasing physical activity without requiring a significant time commitment.

9. Set Reminders

Use reminders on your phone or computer to prompt you to move. These can be set to remind you to stand up, stretch, or take a quick walk at regular intervals throughout the day.

10. Make Movement a Habit

Incorporate movement into your daily routines until it becomes a habit. This could mean performing calf raises while brushing your teeth or doing gentle stretching before bed. The goal is to make physical activity a natural part of your daily life.

Chapter 7:

Addressing Common Ailments and Diseases

Colds and Flu

Colds and flu are among the most common infectious diseases affecting humans, with millions of cases reported annually worldwide. While both are respiratory illnesses, they are caused by different viruses and can have varying levels of severity. In this section, based on Barbara O'Neill's teachings, we explore natural approaches to prevent and manage these ailments, emphasizing the body's ability to heal itself through proper care and support.

Understanding Colds and Flu

Colds are caused by numerous viruses, with rhinoviruses being the most common. Symptoms typically include a runny or stuffy nose, sore throat, coughing, and sneezing. Flu, on the other hand, is caused by influenza viruses and can lead to more severe symptoms, including high fever, body aches, extreme tiredness, and dry cough. Prevention and early intervention are key to managing these illnesses.

Prevention Strategies

- Strengthen the Immune System: A strong immune system can ward off viruses more effectively. Eating a nutrient-rich diet, getting enough sleep, managing stress, and engaging in regular physical activity are fundamental to maintaining immune health.
- Hygiene Practices: Regular hand washing with soap and water, avoiding close contact with sick individuals, and covering the mouth and nose when coughing or sneezing can help prevent the spread of viruses.
- Adequate Nutrition: Consuming foods high in vitamins and minerals, especially vitamin C, vitamin D, zinc, and selenium, can support the immune system's response to infections.

- Stay Hydrated: Drinking plenty of fluids such as water, herbal teas, and broths can help relieve congestion, prevent dehydration, and soothe the respiratory tract.
- Rest: Adequate rest is crucial for recovery. The body heals and regenerates more efficiently when well-rested.
- Warm Soups and Broths: Consuming warm soups and broths can be comforting, help ease congestion, and provide the body with necessary nutrients for recovery.
- Herbal Teas: Teas made from ginger, echinacea, elderberry, and lemon can boost the immune system and alleviate symptoms. Honey, particularly Manuka honey, can be added for its antimicrobial properties and soothing effect on sore throats.
- Steam Inhalation: Inhaling steam can help relieve nasal congestion. Adding essential oils like eucalyptus or peppermint to the water can enhance the decongestant effect.
- Natural Supplements: Vitamin C, vitamin D, zinc, and elderberry supplements have been shown to support the immune system and may reduce the duration and severity of symptoms.
- Garlic: Garlic has natural antimicrobial properties and can support immune function. It can be incorporated into meals or taken as a supplement.

While colds and flu are common, adopting a holistic approach focused on prevention and natural remedies can significantly impact how the body responds to these infections. Strengthening the immune system through a healthy lifestyle, combined with specific natural remedies, can help mitigate symptoms and promote faster recovery. Always consult with a healthcare professional before starting any new treatment, especially if you have underlying health conditions or are pregnant.

Digestive Problems

Digestive problems, ranging from occasional discomfort to chronic conditions, affect millions of people worldwide. These issues can significantly impact quality of life, leading to discomfort, pain, and various health complications. Barbara O'Neill teaches that many digestive problems can be managed or alleviated through natural remedies and lifestyle adjustments, emphasizing the body's inherent ability to heal itself when supported correctly. This section explores natural approaches to addressing common digestive issues, including indigestion, bloating, constipation, and irritable bowel syndrome (IBS).

Understanding Digestive Problems

The digestive system is complex and can be sensitive to diet, stress, and lifestyle factors. Common symptoms of digestive problems include gas, bloating, indigestion, heartburn, constipation, and diarrhea. These issues can stem from a variety of causes, including poor diet, lack of physical activity, stress, and imbalances in gut flora.

Natural Approaches to Digestive Health

- Dietary Changes: The foundation of digestive health is a balanced diet rich in fiber, fruits, vegetables, lean proteins, and healthy fats. Fiber, in particular, is essential for preventing constipation and maintaining a healthy gut microbiome.
- Stay Hydrated: Adequate hydration is crucial for digestion. Water helps break down food, absorb nutrients, and supports regular bowel movements.
- Probiotics and Prebiotics: Probiotics (beneficial bacteria) and prebiotics (food for these bacteria) are vital for gut health. Fermented foods like yogurt, kefir, sauerkraut, and kombucha are excellent sources of probiotics, while prebiotic foods include garlic, onions, bananas, and asparagus.
- Mindful Eating: Eating slowly and mindfully, and chewing food thoroughly, can prevent overeating and indigestion. It allows the digestive system to process food more efficiently, reducing the risk of bloating and discomfort.

- Limit Trigger Foods: Certain foods can exacerbate digestive problems. Common triggers include spicy foods, fatty foods, caffeine, alcohol, and artificial sweeteners. Identifying and avoiding these triggers can significantly improve symptoms.
- Regular Exercise: Physical activity promotes regular bowel movements and can help alleviate symptoms of digestive disorders, such as IBS.
- Stress Management: Stress has a significant impact on digestive health. Techniques such as meditation, yoga, and deep breathing exercises can help manage stress levels and mitigate its effects on the digestive system.
- Herbal Remedies: Various herbs have been traditionally used to aid digestion and relieve discomfort. Peppermint oil, for example, has been shown to alleviate symptoms of IBS, while ginger can reduce nausea and promote gastric emptying.

Digestive health is a crucial aspect of overall well-being. Many digestive problems can be effectively managed through a combination of dietary changes, lifestyle adjustments, and natural remedies. It's important to listen to your body and identify what works best for you, as individual responses to different treatments can vary. If digestive problems persist or worsen, seeking advice from a healthcare professional is recommended to rule out more serious conditions and receive personalized treatment.

Headaches and Migraines

Headaches and migraines are prevalent conditions that affect many people worldwide. While a headache may present as a mild, temporary discomfort, migraines are typically more severe and debilitating, often accompanied by additional symptoms such as sensitivity to light, nausea, and visual disturbances. Barbara O'Neill advocates for a holistic approach to managing these conditions, emphasizing the importance of understanding their triggers and adopting natural remedies and lifestyle changes to mitigate their impact.

Understanding Headaches and Migraines

Headaches can result from a variety of factors, including stress, dehydration, poor posture, eye strain, or underlying health conditions. Migraines, on the other hand, may have genetic roots and are believed to involve changes in brain chemicals and the nervous system. Identifying and managing triggers is a critical step in reducing the frequency and severity of headaches and migraines.

Natural Remedies and Lifestyle Adjustments

- Hydration: Dehydration is a common trigger for headaches. Ensuring adequate fluid intake can prevent the onset of headaches and alleviate symptoms.
- Dietary Modifications: Certain foods and additives, such as aged cheeses, processed foods, MSG, and caffeine, can trigger migraines in some individuals. Keeping a food diary can help identify and eliminate specific dietary triggers.
- Regular Physical Activity: Exercise can reduce the frequency and intensity of headaches and migraines by improving overall health, reducing stress, and promoting regular sleep patterns.
- Stress Management: Stress is a significant trigger for both headaches and migraines. Techniques such as meditation, yoga, deep-breathing exercises, and time management strategies can help manage stress levels.
- Adequate Sleep: Irregular sleep patterns can trigger headaches and migraines. Establishing a regular sleep schedule and creating a restful sleeping environment can improve sleep quality and reduce the likelihood of headaches.
- Essential Oils: Peppermint and lavender essential oils are known for their soothing properties and can be applied topically to the temples or inhaled to relieve headache symptoms.

- Magnesium Supplements: Magnesium deficiency has been linked to migraines. Supplementing with magnesium can help reduce the frequency of migraines in some individuals.
- Herbal Remedies: Feverfew and butterbur are two herbs that have been traditionally used to reduce the frequency and severity of migraine attacks. However, it is essential to consult with a healthcare provider before using these, as they can interact with medications and may not be suitable for everyone.
- Acupuncture: This traditional Chinese medicine technique has been shown to be effective in reducing migraine frequency and severity for some individuals.
- Physical Therapy and Posture Training: For headaches related to tension or poor posture, physical therapy can help alleviate symptoms by improving posture and reducing muscle tension.

Headaches and migraines can significantly impact quality of life, but with the right strategies, their frequency and severity can be managed. By understanding personal triggers and implementing natural remedies and lifestyle changes, individuals can find relief and improve their overall well-being. It's important to consult with healthcare professionals to tailor a treatment plan that addresses individual needs and conditions.

Natural Pain Management Strategies

Pain, whether acute or chronic, is a complex experience that can significantly affect an individual's quality of life. While conventional medicine often relies on pharmaceuticals to manage pain, there is a growing interest in natural and holistic approaches to pain relief. Barbara O'Neill advocates for using natural methods to address the root causes of pain and promote the body's intrinsic healing capabilities. This section explores various natural strategies for managing pain, offering a holistic alternative or complement to conventional pain management techniques.

1. Anti-inflammatory Diet

Diet plays a crucial role in managing inflammation, a common underlying factor in many types of pain. An anti-inflammatory diet emphasizes whole, nutrient-rich foods such as fruits, vegetables, whole grains, nuts, seeds, and omega-3-rich foods like fatty fish. These foods can help reduce inflammation levels in the body, potentially alleviating pain over time.

2. Herbal Remedies

Certain herbs have been shown to have analgesic (pain-relieving) and anti-inflammatory properties. Turmeric, with its active compound curcumin, ginger, willow bark, and Boswellia are among the herbs commonly used to manage pain. These can be taken as supplements, teas, or included in the diet. However, it's essential to consult with a healthcare provider before starting any herbal supplement, especially if taking other medications.

3. Physical Activity and Exercise

Regular physical activity can help reduce pain and improve function, particularly for chronic pain conditions like arthritis and fibromyalgia. Exercise stimulates the release of endorphins, the body's natural painkillers, and helps maintain flexibility and strength. Low-impact activities such as walking, swimming, and yoga are often recommended to start.

4. Acupuncture

Acupuncture is a traditional Chinese medicine technique that involves inserting thin needles into specific points on the body. It is believed to rebalance the body's energy flow (Qi) and has been shown to be effective in treating various types of pain, including headaches, back pain, and osteoarthritis.

5. Massage Therapy

Massage therapy can help relieve pain by reducing muscle tension, improving circulation, and promoting relaxation. It can be particularly beneficial for musculoskeletal pain and tension headaches.

6. Mind-Body Techniques

Techniques that focus on the mind-body connection, such as meditation, mindfulness, and biofeedback, can help individuals manage pain by reducing stress and anxiety, which can exacerbate pain symptoms. These practices can also enhance coping skills, making it easier to live with chronic pain.

7. Hydrotherapy

The use of water for pain relief, known as hydrotherapy, can include baths, showers, water exercises, and cold and hot compresses. The thermal effects of water can help reduce pain and inflammation and promote relaxation.

8. Restorative Sleep

Quality sleep is essential for pain management. Poor sleep can exacerbate pain, creating a vicious cycle. Establishing a regular sleep routine, creating a comfortable sleep environment, and addressing any sleep disorders can improve pain management.

Natural pain management strategies offer a holistic approach to addressing pain, focusing on the whole person rather than just the symptoms. These methods can be used alone or in combination with conventional treatments to provide comprehensive pain management. However, it's important to work with healthcare professionals to develop a personalized pain management plan that considers individual health conditions, preferences, and needs.

Chapter 8:

Specific Remedies for Common Conditions

A-Z Guide to Natural Remedies

This comprehensive A-Z guide provides an overview of natural remedies for a variety of common ailments and health concerns. Drawing from Barbara O'Neill's holistic health principles, this section offers insights into the use of herbs, foods, and lifestyle adjustments to support healing and well-being. It's important to note that while natural remedies can be effective, they should complement traditional medical treatments. Always consult a healthcare professional before trying new remedies, especially if you have existing health conditions or are taking medications.

Aloe Vera

Uses: Burns, skin irritations, digestive health.
Application: Apply gel topically for skin conditions; consume juice for digestive benefits.

Bee Propolis

Uses: Sore throats, immune support.
Application: Throat spray or lozenge form for sore throats; capsules for immune support.

Chamomile

Uses: Anxiety, insomnia, digestive upset.
Application: Drink as tea for relaxation and digestive health.

Dandelion

Uses: Liver detoxification, diuretic.
Application: Consume leaves in salads or drink tea made from roots or leaves.

Echinacea

Uses: Common cold, immune system booster.

Application: Take as tea, tincture, or capsule at the first sign of cold symptoms.

Flaxseed

Uses: High cholesterol, constipation.

Application: Incorporate ground flaxseed into diet for fiber and omega-3 fatty acids.

Ginger

Uses: Nausea, digestive issues, inflammation.

Application: Consume fresh ginger root or take capsules; drink ginger tea.

Honey (Raw)

Uses: Wound healing, coughs, allergies.

Application: Apply topically to wounds; consume for throat soothing and allergy relief.

Iodine (from Kelp)

Uses: Thyroid support.

Application: Consume kelp in food or take kelp supplements for natural iodine.

Jasmine Tea

Uses: Stress relief, antioxidant properties.

Application: Drink tea for relaxation and to support overall health.

Kava

Uses: Anxiety, stress.

Application: Consume as a beverage or supplement; note potential liver toxicity with excessive use.

Lavender

Uses: Stress, insomnia, skin irritations.

Application: Use essential oil for aromatherapy; apply diluted oil topically for skin benefits.

Milk Thistle

Uses: Liver health, detoxification.

Application: Take as a supplement or tea for liver support.

Nettle

Uses: Allergies, inflammation.

Application: Drink as tea or take as a supplement for anti-inflammatory benefits.

Omega-3 Fatty Acids

Uses: Heart health, cognitive function.

Application: Consume fish oil supplements or eat fatty fish regularly.

Peppermint

Uses: Digestive discomfort, headaches.

Application: Drink tea or use essential oil for relief from digestion issues and tension headaches.

Quercetin

Uses: Allergies, inflammation.
Application: Found in onions, apples, and berries; also available as a supplement.

Rosehip

Uses: Vitamin C source, skin health, arthritis relief.
Application: Drink as tea or take as a supplement for its antioxidant properties.

Spirulina

Uses: Energy boost, nutrient-dense supplement.
Application: Add powder to smoothies or take tablets.

Turmeric

Uses: Inflammation, joint pain.
Application: Consume in food, as a tea, or in capsule form; best absorbed with black pepper.

Uva Ursi

Uses: Urinary tract infections.
Application: Take as tea or supplement; note potential for liver damage with long-term use.

Vitamin D

Uses: Bone health, immune support.

Application: Sun exposure, supplements, or vitamin D-rich foods.

Willow Bark

Uses: Pain relief, inflammation.

Application: Take as a tea or supplement; acts as a natural aspirin.

Xylitol

Uses: Dental health.

Application: Use xylitol-sweetened products for reducing cavities and improving oral health.

Yarrow

Uses: Fever, digestive issues.

Application: Drink as tea for its anti-inflammatory and digestive benefits.

Zinc

Uses: Immune support, wound healing.

Application: Consume zinc-rich foods or take supplements to support immune function.

This guide is a starting point for exploring the potential of natural remedies in supporting health and treating common ailments. Remember, the effectiveness of these remedies can vary from person

When to Seek Medical Help

While natural remedies can be effective for managing a range of conditions and promoting overall well-being, it's crucial to recognize when professional medical intervention is necessary. Barbara O'Neill advocates for an informed approach to health, understanding the importance of balancing holistic practices with conventional medical care. This section outlines situations and signs that indicate the need to seek medical help, underscoring the importance of listening to your body and advocating for your health.

Persistent Symptoms

If symptoms persist despite using natural remedies or if they worsen over time, it's important to consult a healthcare professional. Persistent symptoms may indicate an underlying condition that requires medical diagnosis and treatment.

Severe Symptoms

Seek immediate medical attention for severe symptoms such as:

- Difficulty breathing
- Chest pain
- Severe abdominal pain
- High fever
- Sudden and severe headache
- Loss of consciousness or fainting
- Sudden weakness or numbness, especially on one side of the body

Unexplained Weight Loss

Unexpected, significant weight loss without changes in diet or exercise habits can be a sign of an underlying health issue and warrants a medical evaluation.

Chronic Conditions

Individuals with chronic health conditions, such as diabetes, heart disease, or autoimmune disorders, should work closely with healthcare professionals to manage their health, even when incorporating natural remedies into their care plan.

Medication Interactions

Natural remedies, including supplements and herbs, can interact with prescription and over-the-counter medications. Before starting any new remedy, consult a healthcare provider to ensure it's safe and won't interfere with your medications.

Pregnancy and Breastfeeding

Pregnant or breastfeeding women should exercise caution with natural remedies. Many herbs and supplements have not been thoroughly studied for safety during pregnancy and lactation. Always consult with a healthcare provider before using any new treatments during this time.

Children and Elderly

Children and the elderly may have different sensitivities and health needs, making it essential to seek medical advice before introducing new remedies or treatments.

Sudden or Unexplained Symptoms

Sudden or unexplained symptoms, such as a rash, swelling, or dizziness, could indicate an allergic reaction or other urgent health issues. Seek medical attention promptly in these cases.

Understanding when to seek medical help is a crucial aspect of responsible self-care. Natural remedies offer many benefits, but they are part of a broader health management strategy that should include professional medical advice and intervention when necessary. Listening to your body, being mindful of changes in your health, and seeking timely medical care are vital steps in maintaining wellness and ensuring that you receive the most appropriate and effective treatment for your needs.

Chapter 9:

Success Stories

Testimonials from Those Who Have Followed Barbara's Teachings

Throughout her career, Barbara O'Neill has inspired countless individuals to embrace a more holistic approach to health and wellness. Her teachings, which blend scientific knowledge with natural remedies and lifestyle adjustments, have helped many to achieve significant improvements in their health. This chapter showcases testimonials from individuals who have benefited from incorporating Barbara's teachings into their lives, offering personal insights into the transformative power of a natural and mindful approach to health.

Recovery from Chronic Fatigue Syndrome

"For years, I struggled with chronic fatigue syndrome, barely making it through my daily routines. After attending one of Barbara's seminars, I decided to adopt her suggested lifestyle changes, focusing on diet, exercise, and rest. Within months, I noticed a remarkable improvement in my energy levels and overall well-being. It's been a life-changing experience." - Emily R.

Managing Type 2 Diabetes Naturally

"After being diagnosed with type 2 diabetes, I was determined to manage my condition without relying solely on medication. Barbara's advice on diet and natural supplements became my guide. With regular monitoring and adjustments to my lifestyle, I've been able to maintain healthy blood sugar levels and even reduce my medication. I'm grateful for her wisdom." - Mark D.

Overcoming Digestive Issues

"Digestive problems had been a part of my life for as long as I could remember. It wasn't until I stumbled upon Barbara's teachings on digestive health that I found relief.

By following her recommendations on eating whole foods, incorporating probiotics, and managing stress, my digestive system has never been better. Her approach has truly made a difference." - Sarah L.

Relief from Chronic Migraines

"Suffering from chronic migraines was debilitating, affecting my work and personal life. I sought out various treatments with little success until I learned about Barbara O'Neill's holistic approach to health. Implementing her suggestions on diet, hydration, and natural remedies, my migraine frequency and severity have dramatically decreased. It feels like a new lease on life." - Alex G.

Improved Mental Health and Well-being

"Struggling with anxiety and depression, I felt overwhelmed and disconnected. Barbara's teachings on the importance of nutrition, exercise, and mindfulness practices resonated with me. Slowly, I began to incorporate these into my daily life. The improvement in my mental health has been profound, proving to me the power of a holistic approach to well-being." - Jenna K.

These testimonials reflect the wide-ranging impact of Barbara O'Neill's teachings on individuals facing various health challenges. From chronic illnesses to mental health concerns, the adoption of natural remedies, coupled with lifestyle changes, has led to significant health improvements. Barbara's holistic approach underscores the connection between the body, mind, and spirit in achieving overall health and serves as a testament to the healing power of nature and self-care.

How Lifestyle Changes Have Improved Health

This chapter showcases the powerful impact of holistic lifestyle changes on individuals' health, drawing inspiration from Barbara O'Neill's teachings. Through personal testimonials, readers can explore the real-life applications of Barbara's holistic health principles and witness the transformative health benefits achieved by embracing a natural, balanced approach to well-being. These stories serve as compelling evidence of how integrating dietary changes, natural remedies, and lifestyle adjustments can lead to significant improvements in health and quality of life.

Overcoming Digestive Issues

"Before I encountered Barbara's teachings, I suffered from chronic digestive issues, including bloating, discomfort, and irregularity. By adopting a plant-based diet rich in whole foods and incorporating herbal teas and probiotics, I've seen remarkable improvements. Not only have my digestive issues significantly diminished, but I also experience increased energy levels and clearer skin. This journey has taught me the importance of listening to my body and nurturing it with the right foods." - Emma, 34

Managing Chronic Pain Naturally

"Dealing with chronic back pain was an everyday struggle that affected my quality of life. I was reliant on pain medication just to get through the day. Inspired by Barbara's advice on natural pain management, I began practicing yoga and mindfulness meditation, and utilized anti-inflammatory herbs and foods. Gradually, my pain levels decreased, and I gained better control over my condition without solely depending on medication. This holistic approach has not only eased my physical pain but also improved my mental well-being." - David, 42

Reversing Type 2 Diabetes

"After being diagnosed with type 2 diabetes, I feared the impact it would have on my life. However, learning about Barbara O'Neill's approach to health, I decided to make significant lifestyle changes. By adopting a diet low in processed foods and sugars, increasing my physical activity, and monitoring my blood sugar levels naturally, I was able to reverse my diabetes. My doctor was amazed at the improvement in my health markers. This experience has profoundly changed my outlook on health and the power of lifestyle choices." - Luisa, 57

Boosting Immunity and Preventing Illness

"Frequent colds and infections made me realize the importance of a strong immune system. Following Barbara's guidance, I focused on enhancing my immunity through a nutritious diet, regular exercise, and sufficient rest. Additionally, I incorporated immune-supporting supplements like vitamin C, zinc, and echinacea. Since making these changes, I've noticed a significant decrease in the frequency and severity of my illnesses, and I feel more vibrant and resilient." - Michael, 29

Improving Mental Health Through Lifestyle

"Battling anxiety and depression was isolating, but discovering Barbara O'Neill's holistic health principles offered me hope. I embraced regular physical activity, meditation, and a diet rich in omega-3 fatty acids and antioxidants. These lifestyle changes, along with natural remedies and a supportive community, have been instrumental in managing my mental health. I've experienced a noticeable improvement in my mood, stress levels, and overall happiness." - Sophia, 26

These testimonials highlight the profound impact that holistic lifestyle changes can have on various health challenges. By addressing the root causes of health issues, rather than merely treating symptoms, individuals have achieved remarkable improvements in their physical and mental well-being. Barbara O'Neill's teachings remind us of the body's inherent ability to heal and the power of natural approaches in nurturing health and vitality.

Chapter 10:

Building Your Wellness Routine

Creating a Personalized Health Plan

In the journey toward optimal health and well-being, a one-size-fits-all approach is seldom effective. Recognizing this, Barbara O'Neill emphasizes the importance of creating a personalized health plan that addresses individual needs, preferences, and health goals. This chapter guides you through the steps to design your own health plan, inspired by the principles and practices advocated by Barbara, ensuring a balanced and holistic approach to health.

Assess Your Health and Goals

Begin by evaluating your current health status and identifying your wellness goals. Consider factors such as diet, exercise habits, stress levels, sleep quality, and any existing health conditions. Setting clear, achievable goals is crucial, whether it's improving energy levels, managing a health condition, or enhancing overall well-being.

Educate Yourself

Knowledge is power, especially when it comes to health. Invest time in learning about the body's natural healing capabilities, the role of nutrition, the benefits of physical activity, and the importance of mental and emotional well-being. Barbara O'Neill's teachings can be a valuable resource, providing insights into a holistic approach to health.

Dietary Changes

Diet plays a foundational role in health. Tailor your diet to include whole, nutrient-dense foods that support your health goals. Incorporate a variety of fruits, vegetables, whole grains, lean proteins, and healthy fats. Consider any dietary needs specific to your health conditions, and don't hesitate to consult with a nutritionist for personalized advice.

Incorporate Physical Activity

Physical activity is essential for overall health. Design an exercise plan that fits your lifestyle and preferences, ensuring it includes aerobic exercise, strength training, and flexibility exercises. Remember, consistency is more important than intensity; find activities you enjoy to maintain motivation.

Manage Stress

Stress management is a critical component of any health plan. Explore stress-reduction techniques such as meditation, yoga, deep breathing exercises, or spending time in nature. Identify stressors in your life and consider practical steps to minimize their impact.

Prioritize Sleep

Good quality sleep is non-negotiable for health. Establish a regular sleep schedule, create a restful environment, and adopt a calming pre-sleep routine. Address any underlying issues that may be affecting your sleep, such as stress or dietary habits.

Supplementation

While a balanced diet should be your primary source of nutrients, supplements can play a supportive role. Based on your health assessment, consider supplements such as vitamins D and C, omega-3 fatty acids, or probiotics. Always choose high-quality products and consult with a healthcare provider before starting any new supplement.

Monitor Progress and Adjust as Needed

Implement your health plan and monitor your progress towards your goals. Be patient and allow time for changes to manifest. It's important to regularly reassess your plan and make adjustments as needed, based on your experiences and changing health needs.

Seek Professional Guidance

Don't hesitate to seek advice from healthcare professionals, including doctors, nutritionists, and therapists, to support your journey. Their expertise can provide valuable insights and help tailor your health plan to your specific needs.

Creating a personalized health plan is a proactive step towards achieving optimal health and wellness. By integrating the holistic principles championed by Barbara O'Neill, including a balanced diet, regular physical activity, stress management, and sufficient sleep, you can embark on a path that leads to improved health, vitality, and happiness. Remember, the journey to wellness is ongoing, and embracing a holistic approach allows for a fulfilling and healthful life.

Tips for Staying Motivated

Embarking on a journey toward improved health and well-being can be both exciting and challenging. Staying motivated, especially when faced with setbacks or slow progress, is crucial for achieving your health goals. Drawing from the holistic principles of Barbara O'Neill and incorporating wisdom from various health advocates, this section offers practical tips for maintaining motivation and commitment to your personal health plan.

1. Set Realistic Goals

Begin by setting achievable, realistic goals. Whether it's improving your diet, incorporating regular physical activity, or reducing stress, ensure your objectives are specific, measurable, attainable, relevant, and time-bound (SMART). Celebrate small victories along the way to keep yourself motivated.

2. Find Your 'Why'

Understanding your core reasons for wanting to improve your health can provide powerful motivation. Whether it's to enjoy more quality time with loved ones, to achieve a personal challenge, or to live a longer, fuller life, keeping your 'why' in mind can help you stay focused when obstacles arise.

3. Create a Supportive Environment

Surround yourself with supportive people who understand and encourage your health goals. Joining health-focused groups, whether online or in your community, can provide additional motivation and accountability. Sharing your journey with others facing similar challenges can be incredibly uplifting.

4. Track Your Progress

Keeping a journal or log of your progress can be a motivational tool. Documenting what you eat, your physical activity, how you're feeling, and any changes in your health can help you see progress over time, even when it feels slow or invisible.

5. Educate Yourself

Continuously learning about health and wellness can renew your motivation. Reading books, watching documentaries, attending workshops, or listening to podcasts on topics related to your health goals can inspire you and provide new strategies for overcoming challenges.

6. Listen to Your Body

Adopting a holistic approach means listening to your body and respecting its needs. If you're feeling overwhelmed or exhausted, it might be time to reassess your approach. Remember, health is not just about physical fitness or diet; it's also about mental and emotional well-being.

7. Incorporate Variety

Keep your routine interesting by incorporating variety. Trying new healthy recipes, experimenting with different forms of exercise, or exploring new stress-reduction techniques can keep your journey exciting and prevent boredom.

8. Set Up Reminders and Rewards

Use reminders to keep your health goals top of mind, such as setting alarms for exercise or meal planning. Reward yourself for reaching milestones in a way that doesn't undermine your goals, such as a relaxing massage, a new book, or a day trip.

9. Reflect on Your Journey

Regularly take time to reflect on your journey, the progress you've made, and the obstacles you've overcome. This reflection can provide valuable insights into your habits, resilience, and growth, fueling your motivation to continue.

10. Be Patient and Kind to Yourself

Lastly, be patient and kind to yourself. Change takes time, and setbacks are a normal part of any journey. Practice self-compassion, and remind yourself that every step forward, no matter how small, is progress toward a healthier, happier you.

Adapting Barbara's Teachings to Your Life

Incorporating Barbara O'Neill's teachings into your life requires more than just a cursory understanding of her principles; it demands a thoughtful, personalized approach to health and wellness. This section guides you through the process of adapting Barbara's holistic health philosophy to fit your unique circumstances, preferences, and goals. By doing so, you can create a sustainable, enjoyable path to improved health and well-being.

1. Assess Your Starting Point

Begin by taking an honest assessment of your current health status, lifestyle, and habits. Identify areas that align with Barbara's teachings and areas that offer the most significant opportunities for improvement. This might include diet, exercise, stress management, sleep quality, or exposure to natural environments.

2. Prioritize Changes Based on Your Needs

Given the broad spectrum of health and wellness topics covered by Barbara, it's essential to prioritize changes based on your most pressing needs. If you're struggling with dietary issues, focus on nutritional adjustments before tackling other areas. For those battling stress or mental health challenges, techniques for mental and emotional well-being might take precedence.

3. Set Incremental Goals

Implementing a holistic health plan can be overwhelming if you attempt to change everything at once. Instead, set incremental, achievable goals that gradually align your lifestyle more closely with Barbara's teachings. Small, consistent changes are more sustainable and less daunting, leading to long-term success.

4. Customize Solutions to Fit Your Life

Barbara's teachings provide a framework, but they are not one-size-fits-all. Customize her advice to fit your personal preferences, lifestyle, and circumstances. This might mean adapting recipes to suit your dietary restrictions, finding physical activities that you enjoy, or fitting in mindfulness practices amidst a busy schedule.

5. Integrate Mind-Body-Spirit Connection

At the core of Barbara's philosophy is the integration of mind, body, and spirit. Look for ways to nurture each aspect of your being. This holistic approach ensures that you're not just focusing on physical health but also attending to your mental, emotional, and spiritual well-being.

6. Learn Continuously

Barbara's teachings encourage ongoing learning and self-discovery. Stay curious and open to new information, research, and techniques that can enhance your health journey. This might involve reading books, attending workshops, or connecting with like-minded individuals who share your commitment to holistic health.

7. Practice Patience and Persistence

Adapting to a new health philosophy takes time, and results may not be immediate. Practice patience and persistence, understanding that health and wellness are lifelong journeys. Celebrate your progress, learn from setbacks, and stay committed to your goals.

8. Seek Support and Community

Embarking on this journey can be more enriching and less challenging with support from others who share your values and goals. Seek out communities, both online and in-person, where you can find encouragement, share experiences, and learn from others following Barbara's teachings.

9. Reflect and Adjust Regularly

Regularly reflect on your journey, acknowledging your achievements and reassessing your goals as your needs and circumstances change. Being flexible and willing to adjust your approach will help you stay aligned with your health and wellness objectives over the long term.

10. Embrace Holistic Health as a Lifestyle

Finally, understand that adapting Barbara's teachings to your life is not about following a strict set of rules; it's about embracing holistic health as a lifestyle. This means making conscious choices every day that contribute to your overall well-being, leading to a healthier, happier, and more balanced life

Glossary of Terms

This glossary provides definitions for terms and concepts related to holistic health, natural remedies, and wellness as discussed throughout the book. Understanding these terms will help readers better grasp the principles of Barbara O'Neill's teachings and apply them more effectively in their pursuit of a healthier lifestyle.

1. Antioxidants: Substances that protect the body's cells from damage caused by free radicals. Common antioxidants include vitamins C and E, selenium, and carotenoids, which are found in many fruits and vegetables.

2. Bioavailability: The rate and extent to which a nutrient is absorbed and used by the body. Factors such as food preparation and individual health can influence nutrient bioavailability.

3. Detoxification (Detox): The process by which the body eliminates toxins and waste materials. Detoxification can be supported by certain foods, herbs, and lifestyle practices.

4. Fermentation: A metabolic process that produces chemical changes in organic substrates through the action of enzymes. In food, fermentation can enhance nutritional value, create beneficial enzymes, and promote the growth of probiotics.

5. Free Radicals: Unstable molecules that can damage cells, contributing to aging and diseases. Free radicals are generated by natural body processes and environmental exposures.

6. Holistic Health: An approach to life and wellness that considers the whole person, including their physical, mental, emotional, and spiritual well-being, rather than just focusing on specific symptoms or diseases.

7. Homeostasis: The body's ability to maintain stable internal conditions (such as temperature and pH levels) despite changes in the external environment.

8. Inflammation: A natural process by which the body's immune system responds to injury or infection. While necessary for healing, chronic inflammation is linked to various health conditions, including heart disease and arthritis.

9. Macronutrients: Nutrients that the body needs in large amounts to maintain health and provide energy. The three main macronutrients are carbohydrates, proteins, and fats.

10. Micronutrients: Essential vitamins and minerals that the body needs in smaller amounts for various functions, including growth, disease prevention, and well-being.

11. Phytochemicals: Natural compounds found in plants that have beneficial effects on health. Phytochemicals can have antioxidant, anti-inflammatory, and anti-cancer properties.

12. Probiotics: Live microorganisms that, when consumed in adequate amounts, confer a health benefit on the host. Probiotics are found in fermented foods like yogurt, kefir, and sauerkraut.

13. Whole Foods: Foods that are minimally processed or refined and are free from additives or other artificial substances. Whole foods include fruits, vegetables, whole grains, nuts, and seeds.

14. Mindfulness: A practice of being fully present and engaged in the moment, aware of one's thoughts, feelings, bodily sensations, and surrounding environment, without judgment.

15. Hydrotherapy: The use of water in various forms and temperatures for health and healing purposes, including baths, steam, and ice.

Understanding these terms is essential for navigating the world of holistic health and making informed decisions about personal health and wellness practices.

Summary of Key Principles

In the book, we've explored the comprehensive teachings of Barbara O'Neill on achieving health and well-being through natural means. This summary encapsulates the key principles outlined throughout the book, serving as a concise guide to the core tenets of Barbara's holistic health philosophy.

1. Whole Foods Diet: Emphasize a diet rich in whole, plant-based foods that are minimally processed. This includes a variety of fruits, vegetables, whole grains, nuts, and seeds. Such a diet provides essential nutrients, fiber, and antioxidants, supporting overall health and preventing chronic diseases.

2. Hydration: Drink plenty of clean, pure water daily. Proper hydration is crucial for maintaining the body's functions, including digestion, circulation, and toxin elimination.

3. Physical Activity: Incorporate regular physical exercise into your routine. Exercise improves cardiovascular health, boosts the immune system, enhances mood, and helps manage weight.

4. Sunlight: Seek sensible sun exposure to maintain adequate vitamin D levels, which are vital for bone health, immune function, and mood regulation.

5. Fresh Air and Nature: Spend time outdoors in fresh air and natural surroundings. Being in nature has been shown to reduce stress, enhance mood, and improve mental health.

6. Rest and Sleep: Ensure you get enough quality sleep and rest. Sleep is essential for healing, rejuvenation, and maintaining cognitive function and emotional health.

7. Stress Management: Adopt stress-reduction techniques such as meditation, yoga, deep breathing, or mindfulness. Managing stress is key to preventing a range of health issues, including heart disease and anxiety.

8. Avoid Toxins: Minimize exposure to toxins in food, water, air, and personal care products. Choose organic where possible, and use natural cleaning and personal care products.

9. Natural Remedies: Utilize the healing power of herbs and natural supplements to support health and treat ailments. Always seek advice from a healthcare professional before starting any new supplement.

10. Emotional and Spiritual Well-being: Foster a positive outlook on life and nurture your spiritual health through practices that resonate with you, such as prayer, meditation, or spending time with loved ones.

11. Education and Self-empowerment: Continuously educate yourself about health and wellness. Being informed empowers you to make choices that are best for your health and well-being.

12. Community and Support: Build a supportive community around you. Sharing your journey with like-minded individuals can provide encouragement, motivation, and accountability.

By integrating these principles into your daily life, you embark on a path toward natural wellness, aligning with Barbara O'Neill's vision of health that is holistic, balanced, and sustainable. Remember, the journey to health is a personal one, filled with discoveries and growth along the way.

Encouragement for the Journey Towards Health

Embarking on the journey towards better health, inspired by the teachings of Barbara O'Neill, is a commendable step toward self-improvement and holistic well-being. This path, while immensely rewarding, may present challenges and require perseverance. Herein lies encouragement and guidance to support you through this transformative process.

Believe in Your Ability to Change

The first and perhaps most crucial step is to believe in your own capacity for change. Your body is a remarkable system, capable of healing and regeneration, given the right conditions. Trust in this innate ability and know that every positive choice you make is a step towards better health.

Embrace the Journey

View this journey not as a temporary phase but as a lifelong commitment to yourself. There will be successes and setbacks, but each experience offers valuable lessons. Celebrate your progress, no matter how small, and learn from the challenges without judgment.

Patience is Key

True health and wellness are not achieved overnight. It takes time to undo habits and see the full benefits of your efforts. Be patient with yourself and the process. Remember, incremental changes can lead to significant health transformations over time.

Seek Support

You are not alone in this journey. Seek out communities and individuals who share your commitment to natural health and wellness. Sharing your experiences, challenges, and successes with others can provide encouragement, motivation, and accountability.

Stay Informed

Knowledge is a powerful tool on your path to health. Continue to educate yourself about holistic health principles, natural remedies, and healthy lifestyle practices. However, always consider the source of your information and consult healthcare professionals when necessary.

Listen to Your Body

Your body is an excellent communicator, offering clues about what it needs to thrive. Pay attention to how different foods, activities, and lifestyle choices affect you physically and emotionally. Use this feedback to fine-tune your approach to health and well-being.

Find Joy in the Process

Integrate practices that bring you joy and fulfillment. Whether it's cooking a nutritious meal, engaging in physical activity you love, or practicing mindfulness, these should be sources of happiness rather than obligations.

Commit to Self-Care

Prioritize self-care as an essential component of your health journey. This encompasses not just diet and exercise, but also stress management, sleep, and activities that nourish your soul.

Reflect and Adjust

Regularly reflect on your journey, acknowledging how far you've come and where you'd like to go. Be open to adjusting your approach as your health needs and life circumstances change.

Spread the Knowledge

As you learn and grow, share your knowledge and experiences with others. Your journey could inspire someone else to embark on their path to health and wellness.

A Final Note of Encouragement

Remember, the journey to health is deeply personal and uniquely yours. It's about finding balance, harmony, and joy in ways that respect your body's needs and your life's circumstances. Armed with the teachings of Barbara O'Neill and a commitment to yourself, you have everything you need to achieve lasting health and wellness. Here's to your health, happiness, and the vibrant life that awaits you on this journey.

Conclusion

As we reach the conclusion of our journey, it's important to reflect on the profound teachings of Barbara O'Neill and the impact they can have on our lives. This book has not only introduced us to the principles of holistic health and natural remedies but also guided us on how to incorporate these teachings into our daily routines to achieve a balanced and healthy lifestyle.

Barbara O'Neill's approach, grounded in the understanding that the body is an incredibly sophisticated entity capable of healing itself given the right conditions, invites us to re-evaluate our relationship with our bodies, our health, and the natural world. From the importance of a plant-based, whole-food diet to the benefits of physical activity, sunlight, fresh air, and water, each chapter has provided actionable insights to empower us on our health journey.

We've explored how simple lifestyle changes can have profound effects on our well-being, reducing our risk of chronic diseases, enhancing our mental health, and improving our overall quality of life. The personal testimonials shared in this book serve as a testament to the transformative power of adopting a holistic approach to health, echoing the success stories of those who have walked this path before us.

As you close this book, remember that the journey to optimal health is a personal and ongoing process. It's about making conscious decisions every day that align with your well-being. The teachings of Barbara O'Neill offer a foundation upon which you can build a healthier, more vibrant life, but it's your commitment, motivation, and perseverance that will turn these principles into lasting habits.

Let this book be a resource you return to time and again, not just for its natural remedies and health advice, but as a source of inspiration and encouragement. The path to wellness is not always linear, and challenges are an inevitable part of growth. However, with each small step, you're investing in your most valuable asset—your health.

In the end, embracing Barbara O'Neill's teachings is about more than just improving your physical health; it's about nurturing a sense of harmony and balance in all aspects of your life. It's a journey of discovery, learning, and ultimately, transformation.

Thank you for allowing us to be a part of your journey to natural wellness. Here's to your health, happiness, and a life lived in harmony with nature's wisdom.

Made in the USA
Las Vegas, NV
18 May 2024

90053552R10057